CORE EXERCISES FOR SENIORS OVER 60

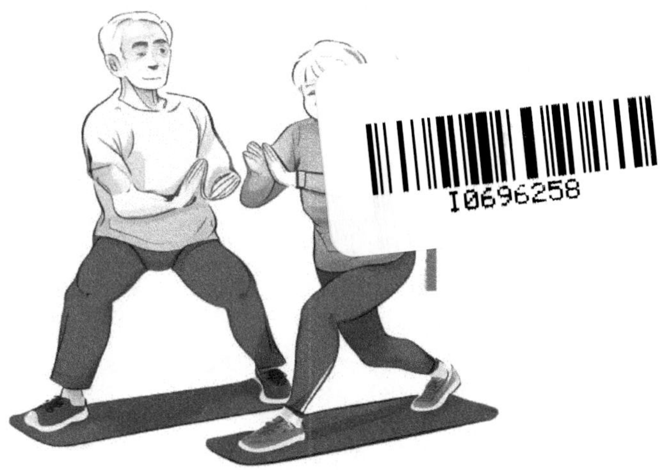

Effective Daily Workout Routine to Boost Energy and Build Balance for the Aged or Elderly over Sixty

DR. BRENDA GRIMM

TABLE OF CONTENT

INTRODUCTION

My aged mum had been struggling with mobility issues for years. As an active senior, she was determined to get her strength back, so she picked up this book, titled **"Core Exercises for Seniors over 60"**. At first, she was daunted by the length and complexity of the exercises, but she read through this book thoroughly and was committed to following the program.

After a few weeks, she started to feel the impact of the exercises as her mobility improved and she was able to do everyday tasks with much more ease. Her newfound strength and agility surprised even her, and she was soon able to take on activities she had not done in years. She was so proud of her achievement, and she attributed it all to the exercise routine she had read and followed in my book.

Welcome to Core Exercises for Seniors! This book is designed to help keep seniors over the age of 60 in shape and feeling great. Core exercises are an essential part of any fitness routine, and this book will help you get started with a safe and effective core exercise routine.

We will discuss the importance of core exercises, the best exercises to perform, and how to create a weekly schedule that will keep you motivated and engaged.

Core exercises are an essential part of a balanced fitness routine. They help strengthen the muscles in the abdomen, back, and pelvis, which are vital for overall strength, stability, and balance. Core exercises also help improve posture, reduce injury risk, and improve overall fitness levels.

With regular practice, seniors over the age of 60 can enjoy the many benefits of a strong and healthy core. In this book, we will discuss the best core exercises for seniors over 60, and how to create a weekly schedule that will keep you motivated and engaged.

We will also discuss the importance of proper form and breathing when performing core exercises, as well as tips for making the exercises more challenging as you progress.

With this book, you will have all the information you need to create a safe and effective core exercise routine that will help you stay in shape and feeling great.

CHAPTER 1

THE EFFECTIVE POWER OF YOUR CORE

In our society, we often take for granted the importance of our core. Our core is what allows us to stand upright, maintain balance, and move with grace. As we age, the strength and stability of our core become essential to our well-being and independence.

In this chapter, we will explore the powerful effects of strengthening our core and how it can improve our overall quality of life. The core is a complex system of muscles that form a ring around the midsection of our body.

It is comprised of the abdominal and back muscles, along with the hips and pelvic floor. When these muscles are strong and stable, we are able to move with better balance and coordination.

Additionally, strong core muscles provide support for our organs and helps us to maintain good posture.

This is especially important for seniors over 60, as poor posture can lead to chronic pain and other mobility issues. The core is also important for balance and stability. Strong core muscles provide support for our spine, which can help us to remain upright and reduce the risk of falls.

A strong core can also help us to move gracefully and with ease, reducing the risk of accidental slips and falls. When it comes to core exercises, there are a variety of options available for seniors over 60.

Some of the most beneficial exercises are those that are low-impact and focus on building strength and stability. These can include exercises such as planks, bridges, and side planks. Yoga and Pilates can also be beneficial, as they can help to strengthen the core while also improving flexibility and balance.

There are also a variety of other exercises that can help to improve the strength and stability of our core muscles. These can include squats, lunges, and abdominal exercises such as crunches and sit-ups.

While these exercises are beneficial, seniors over 60 should always consult their doctor before beginning any new exercise program.

The effective power of a strong and stable core can be truly remarkable. Not only can it improve our posture and balance, but it can also help to reduce the risk of falls and other mobility issues.

A strong core can also help us to move with ease and grace, allowing us to maintain our independence and enjoy a higher quality of life.

By incorporating core exercises into our daily routine, seniors over 60 can experience the powerful benefits of a strong and stable core.

I.   What Is Your Core?

The core is the foundation of your body, and it is responsible for your posture, balance, and overall stability. It is made up of a group of muscles located in the center of the body, including the abdominal muscles, lower back muscles, and the pelvic floor muscles.

These muscles work together to maintain your posture and stability while performing everyday activities. The core muscles are the powerhouse of your body. They provide stability and balance, as well as enabling you to perform a range of movements.

The core muscles help to support your spine, which is integral in preventing injuries from occurring. Additionally, the core muscles are important for balance and stability, as well as helping to control the movements of your arms and legs.

The core muscles are also important for posture. They help to maintain the natural curve of your spine and provide an anchor for the shoulder and hip muscles. This helps to keep your body in an upright, balanced position, which reduces fatigue and strain on the body.

Strong core muscles are essential for seniors over 60 to reduce the risk of falls and injuries. Core exercises are an effective way to build strength and stability in the core muscles.

Core exercises also help to improve balance and coordination, as well as increasing overall strength and flexibility. Core exercises can be done at home or at the gym and are designed to target the core muscles in a safe and effective way.

In conclusion, the core is a vital muscle group for seniors over 60. Core exercises can help to strengthen and stabilize the core muscles, reduce the risk of falls and injuries, and improve overall posture and balance.

II. Aging in Relation to Your Body

Aging is a natural part of life, but that doesn't mean it has to be a bad thing. As you age, it's important to understand how your body is changing and how you can best take care of it.

As you get older, it's important to understand that your body is no longer the same as when you were younger and it's important to adjust your physical activity to accommodate the changes. Your core muscles, which are a group of muscles located in your abdomen, are usually the first to show signs of aging.

As you age, these muscles weaken, making it more difficult to perform activities that require strength and balance. This is why it's so important to focus on strengthening your core muscles and keeping them active as you age.

One of the best ways to do this is to begin a regular core exercise routine. Core exercises are great for strengthening your core muscles and improving your balance and stability.

Core exercises can help you maintain the strength of your core muscles, which can help you stay active and mobile.

Core exercises can also help you improve your posture, which can reduce pain and discomfort as you age. It's also important to remember that as you age, your body needs more rest and recovery.

Make sure you are getting enough rest and taking the time to properly stretch and warm up before any activity. Taking care of your body as you age can help you stay active and healthy for years to come.

Overall, aging can be a difficult process, but it doesn't have to be. With proper care and maintenance of your body, you can stay active and healthy well into your golden years.

Understanding the changes your body is going through and how to best take care of it can help you live a healthy and active lifestyle for years to come. Focusing on core exercises for seniors over 60 can help you maintain the strength of your core muscles and live a healthy and active life.

III. The Threatening Factors of a Weak Core You Didn't Know About

A crucial component of the human body is the core. It is composed of the muscles, ligaments, and tendons that make up the abdominal, back, and hip regions. As people age, their core strength tends to decline, making them more prone to injury and falls.

This is why it is important for seniors over 60 to maintain a strong core. However, there are a number of threatening factors that can make a weak core more dangerous.

The first of these factors is poor posture. Poor posture can lead to a variety of issues, including back pain and muscle imbalances. Poor posture also places extra stress on the core muscles, which can lead to further weakening over time.

Seniors should make sure they are sitting and standing with good posture, and should practice exercises that strengthen their core muscles in order to help reduce the strain on their bodies.

Another factor that can lead to a weak core is a lack of exercise. As people age, their activity levels tend to decrease due to physical limitations and a decrease in motivation. This can cause the core muscles to weaken, leading to a decrease in stability and balance.

To combat this, seniors should make an effort to stay active, incorporating strength training and balance exercises into their routine. In addition to a lack of exercise, a weak core can also be caused by poor nutrition.

As people age, their bodies need more nutrients in order to maintain muscle strength. Without proper nutrition, their core muscles can become weak, putting them at risk for falls and other injuries.

Seniors should make sure they are eating a balanced diet and taking any necessary supplements in order to ensure their bodies are getting the nutrients they need.

Finally, a weak core can be caused by medical conditions. Many medical conditions, such as arthritis and osteoporosis, can cause the core muscles to weaken.

In addition, certain medications can lead to muscle loss, including those used to treat high blood pressure and diabetes. Seniors should speak to their doctor about any concerns they may have in order to ensure they are getting the best treatment possible.

In conclusion, weak core muscles can be a very dangerous condition for seniors over 60. Poor posture, lack of exercise, poor nutrition, and medical conditions can all contribute to a weak core.

To ensure their safety and prevent injury, seniors should make sure they are taking steps to maintain a strong core, including getting regular exercise, eating a balanced diet, and discussing any medical concerns they may have with their doctor.

IV. The Healthy Benefits of Strengthening Your Core Your Doctor Didn't Disclose to You

When it comes to improving your overall health and well-being, strengthening your core is essential. The core muscles in your body are the foundation for all movement and provide stability, balance, and support for your entire body.

Strengthening your core muscles can have a number of positive effects on your physical, mental, and emotional health. Strengthening your core can help you become more flexible and agile.

Core exercises can help you improve your posture, balance, coordination, and body awareness. This can help you move more efficiently and reduce the risk of injuries.

Core exercises also help to build strength in your back and abdominal muscles, which can help to support your spine and reduce back pain.

Strengthening your core muscles can also help to improve your overall physical fitness.

Core exercises can increase your heart rate and help you burn more calories during a workout. They can also improve your muscular endurance and help to build muscle mass.

This can help you increase your physical strength and give you the energy you need to exercise for longer periods of time. Strengthening your core can also have positive effects on your mental and emotional health.

Core exercises can help to reduce stress and anxiety, improve your mood, and boost your self-confidence.

They can also help you build strength, which can help to give you a sense of accomplishment and satisfaction.

Strengthening your core can also help to support your internal organs and improve digestion. Core exercises can help to stimulate your digestive system, increase your metabolism, and help to flush out toxins from your body.

This can help to improve your overall health and prevent a variety of illnesses. Overall, strengthening your core can have a number of positive benefits for your physical, mental, and emotional health.

Core exercises can help to improve your flexibility, posture, balance, coordination, and body awareness. They can also help to improve your physical fitness, reduce stress and anxiety, and support your internal organs.

Strengthening your core can be an important part of maintaining a healthy lifestyle and can help to improve your overall well-being.

Motivational Exercise Quote

Age is just a number;

Your determination is the real measure of your strength.

Keep moving, keep thriving.

CHAPTER 2

DEVELOPING A ROCK-SOLID CORE

Developing a rock-solid core is a critical aspect of any fitness program. A strong core provides stability and can improve posture, balance, and overall performance.

It is especially important for seniors over 60 to maintain a strong core, as this can help reduce the risk of falls and other injuries. The core is made up of numerous muscle groups, including the abdominal muscles, lower back muscles, pelvic floor muscles, and hip flexors.

It is important to target all of these muscles when developing a rock-solid core. Fortunately, there are a variety of exercises that can help achieve this.

Exercises that Can Help Build a Rock-solid Core

- First, the abdominal muscles should be targeted. Exercises like the plank and side plank can help strengthen the core and improve posture.

  To do a plank, start in a push-up position with the arms straight and the body in a straight line from the head to the toes. Hold for 10-30 seconds, then lower the body down to the forearms, and hold for 10-30 seconds.

  To do a side plank, start on the side with the feet stacked and the elbow and forearm supporting the body. After holding for 10 to 30 seconds, switch sides.

- Second, the lower back muscles should be targeted. Exercises like the bridge and cat-cow can help strengthen the lower back and improve posture.

To do a bridge, start lying on the back with the knees bent and feet flat on the floor. Squeeze the glutes and lift the hips up, hold for 10-30 seconds, then slowly lower the hips back down.

To do a cat-cow, start on all fours with the hands and knees on the floor. Take a deep breath, arching the back and lifting the head, then exhale and round the back, tucking the chin. Repeat 10-15 times.

- Third, the pelvic floor muscles should be targeted. Exercises like the kegel and hip bridge can help strengthen the pelvic floor muscles.

To do a kegel, sit or lie down, and slowly squeeze and lift the pelvic floor muscles. Then, gradually release after holding for 10 to 30 seconds.

To do a hip bridge, start lying on the back with the knees bent and feet flat on the floor. Squeeze the glutes and lift the hips up, hold for 10-30 seconds, then slowly lower the hips back down.

- Finally, the hip flexors should be targeted. Exercises like the hip flexor stretch and single-leg bridge can help strengthen the hip flexors.

To do a hip flexor stretch, start in a lunge position with the back knee bent and the front knee at a 90-degree angle. Switch sides after holding for 10 to 30 seconds.

To do a single-leg bridge, start lying on the back with one knee bent and the other leg lifted straight up. Squeeze the glutes and lift the hips up, hold for 10-30 seconds, then slowly lower the hips back down.

To develop a rock-solid core, these exercises should be done 2-3 times a week. It is important to start slowly, with low intensity, and work up to higher intensity as the core muscles become stronger.

Additionally, it is important to focus on proper form and breath control to ensure the exercises are being done correctly and safely.

In conclusion, developing a rock-solid core is an important part of any fitness program. For seniors over 60, it is especially important, as it can help reduce the risk of falls and other injuries.

There are a variety of exercises that can help achieve this, including the plank, bridge, cat-cow, kegel, hip flexor stretch, and single-leg bridge.

It is important to start slowly, with low intensity, and work up to higher intensity as the core muscles become stronger.

With dedication and consistency, a strong and stable core can be achieved.

I. How to Exercise Your Core

Exercising your core is an essential part of staying physically fit and healthy as you age. A strong core provides stability and support for your body, helping to reduce the risk of falls and injuries.

Core exercises are also important for improving balance, posture and flexibility, which are all important for staying active and independent.

The core muscles are the muscles in your abdomen, lower back, and hips that support your spine and body. These muscles help you to balance, move and twist, and work together to maintain posture and protect your spine.

To begin, start by standing up tall and engaging your abdominal muscles by drawing your belly button in towards your spine. This will help to activate your core muscles and prepare them for the exercises you'll be doing.

 The first exercise to try is the plank. Begin on your knees and hands, placing your knees precisely behind your hips and your hands under your shoulders.

Engage your abdominal muscles and slowly lift your knees off the floor, keeping your body in a straight line and your hips level. Hold this position for as long as you can, up to one minute if possible.

As you become stronger, try to increase the length of time you hold the plank. Another great exercise for your core is the bridge.

Laying on your back with your knees bent and your feet flat on the floor is the best position to begin this exercise.

Engage your core muscles, and slowly lift your hips off the floor. Hold this position for a few seconds, and then slowly lower your hips back to the floor.

With this workout, try to perform 10 to 15 repetitions. Your core muscles will benefit greatly from the bird dog workout. Begin on your knees and hands, placing your knees precisely behind your hips and your hands under your shoulders.

Engage your abdominal muscles and extend your right arm in front of you and your left leg behind you. Hold the position for a few seconds and then alternate to the other side. With this workout, try to do 10 to 15 repetitions.

Another great core exercise is the Superman. To do this exercise, start by lying on your stomach, with your arms extended in front of you and your legs extended behind you. Engage your abdominal muscles and raise your arms and legs off the ground as high as you can.

Hold this position for a few seconds, and then slowly lower your arms and legs back to the floor. Aim to do 10-15 repetitions of this exercise.

Finally, the seated twist is an effective exercise for strengthening your core muscles. Sit in a chair with your feet flat on the floor to begin this exercise.

Engage your abdominal muscles and twist your upper body to one side. Maintain this position for a little while, then shift back to your starting position.

Alternate sides, and aim to do 10-15 repetitions of this exercise.

Exercising your core is an important part of staying healthy and active as you age. By incorporating these exercises into your routine, you can help to reduce the risk of falls and injuries, and improve your balance, posture and flexibility.

Have fun and be sure to listen to your body while you exercise.

II. The Appropriate Environment to Exercise

Exercising regularly is an important part of any senior's routine and can help improve strength, balance, and flexibility. But for seniors over 60, the environment in which you choose to exercise is just as important as the exercises themselves.

It's important to create an environment that is safe and supportive so you can maximize your fitness goals. The first thing to consider when creating an appropriate environment for exercise is the type of activity being performed.

Different activities require different environments. For example, if you're planning to do anaerobic workout such as running, you'll need an open space with a flat, even surface.

On the other hand, if you're planning to do weight training, you'll need a space that is large enough to accommodate the equipment and has a flat, non-slip surface. When selecting a space, it's important to consider your safety and the safety of those around you.

The second important factor to consider is lighting. This is particularly important if you're exercising outdoors. Make sure the area is well-lit, especially if you're exercising in the early morning or evening hours.

If you're exercising indoors, make sure the lighting is adequate for the activity you're doing. You should also be aware of any overhead lights which can cause glare and make it difficult to see.

The temperature of the environment is also important. High temperatures can cause dehydration and heat exhaustion, while low temperatures can cause hypothermia and frostbite.

Try to find a space with a comfortable temperature, and if necessary, use fans or air conditioning to keep the area cool. If you're exercising outdoors, try to find an area that is shaded to provide relief from the sun.

The fourth factor to consider is sound. Loud music can be distracting and can make it difficult to focus on the task at hand. If you're exercising outdoors, be aware of any background noise such as traffic or construction.

If you're exercising indoors, try to keep the volume of music or television at a level that won't interfere with your concentration.

Finally, if you're exercising at home, make sure the area is free of any obstacles that could cause you to trip or slip. Remove any loose cords, rugs, or furniture that could present a tripping hazard.

Make sure the space is clean and clear of any clutter, and consider covering any hard surfaces with a rubberized exercise mat. Creating a safe, supportive environment is essential for seniors over 60 who are serious about exercising.

Consider the type of activity you'll be doing, the lighting, temperature, sound, and any potential hazards that may be present. With the right environment, you can maximize your fitness goals and stay safe and healthy.

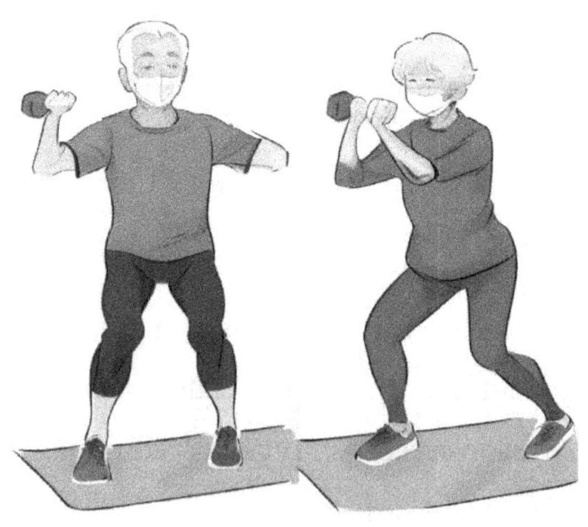

III. Exercising at the right time to achieve the Best Result

When it comes to exercising, timing is everything. Knowing when to exercise can be the difference between achieving your goals and falling short.

Exercise can be a great way to improve your health, strength, and overall well-being, but if done at the wrong times, it can be ineffective. Exercising at the wrong time can cause fatigue, muscle strain, and even injury.

This is especially true for seniors over 60. Seniors have to be especially mindful about when they choose to exercise. With the right timing, seniors can achieve optimal results from their workouts.

The first thing to consider when deciding when to exercise is your own energy levels. Everyone has a different energy level throughout the day. Some people feel more energized in the morning, while others may prefer to exercise in the afternoon or at night.

It is important to find the time of day that works best for you and your energy levels.

The next thing to consider is the type of exercise you are doing. Different exercises require different levels of intensity and exertion. For example, a high-intensity workout such as running or weight training should be done when you are feeling the most energized.

On the other hand, low-intensity exercises such as stretching or yoga can be done at any time of the day. It's also important to factor in rest days.

Rest days are essential for muscle recovery and preventing injury. Make sure to give your body adequate time to rest and recover between workouts. This will help you achieve the best results without putting too much strain on your body.

Finally, it is important to find a balance between exercise and other activities. Exercise should not be the only activity that you do throughout the day.

Make sure to include other activities such as reading, socializing, and relaxing in your daily routine. This will help keep you energized and motivated to exercise.

Overall, the best time to exercise is when you feel the most energized and have adequate time to rest and recover. This will ensure that you get the most out of your workouts and achieve the best results.

With the right timing, seniors can improve their health, strength, and overall well-being.

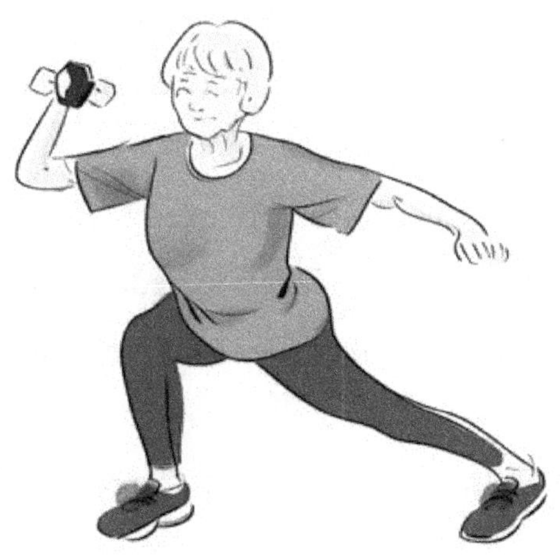

IV. Controllable Mistakes to Avoid While Exercising

The goal of any core exercise program is to build a strong and healthy core, while avoiding common mistakes that can lead to injury. So, if you are a senior over 60 and embarking on a core exercise routine, here are some of the most common mistakes to avoid in order to achieve the best results.

1. **Not Warming Up and Cooling Down:** Before starting any core exercise routine, it is important to warm up your muscles. Warming up helps to prepare the muscles for exercise and can prevent injuries.

    When finished with core exercises, cooling down is also important. It helps to reduce muscle soreness and can help reduce the risk of injuries.

2. **Not Doing the Exercises Correctly:** When doing core exercises, it is vital to do them correctly. Improper form can lead to muscle strain, which can cause pain and soreness.

To ensure that you are doing the exercises correctly, make sure you have a qualified professional demonstrating the movements.

3. **Overdoing it:** It is easy to become too enthusiastic and do too much too soon. This can lead to soreness and fatigue. To avoid this, start slowly and gradually increase the intensity of your workouts.

4. **Not Listening to Your Body:** It is important to listen to your body and recognize when it needs a break. When you start to feel pain or fatigue, it is best to stop and rest. Overworking your core can lead to injuries that may take a long time to heal.

5. **Not Eating Right:** Eating a balanced diet with plenty of fresh fruits and vegetables is important. Eating a healthy diet will help to ensure that your body has the nutrients it needs to exercise and recover properly.

6. **Not Stretching:** Stretching is an important part of any core exercise program. It helps to reduce muscle soreness and injury. Before and after each workout, make sure to stretch your core muscles to ensure that they remain flexible.

7. **Not Paying Attention to Posture:** Good posture is important in any core exercise program. Slouching or hunching over can reduce the effectiveness of the exercises and can lead to injury. Make sure to keep your back straight and your shoulders back when doing core exercises.

8. **Not Incorporating Variety:** Doing the same core exercises day after day can become boring and can lead to a plateau in your progress. To avoid this, try to incorporate a variety of exercises such as planks, crunches, sit-ups, and other core exercises.

9. **Not Taking Time to Rest:** Rest is an important part of any fitness routine. Make sure to give your core muscles time to recover after each workout. This will help to reduce the risk of injury and fatigue.

10. **Not Setting Realistic Goals:** It is important to set realistic goals for yourself. Don't expect to be able to do a full plank if you are just starting out. Set achievable goals and gradually progress towards more difficult exercises.

By avoiding these common mistakes, you can ensure that you get the most out of your core exercise program.

Remember, in order to get the best results, you will need to be consistent, listen to your body, and take the time to warm up and cool down. With patience and dedication, you can achieve a rock-solid core in no time!

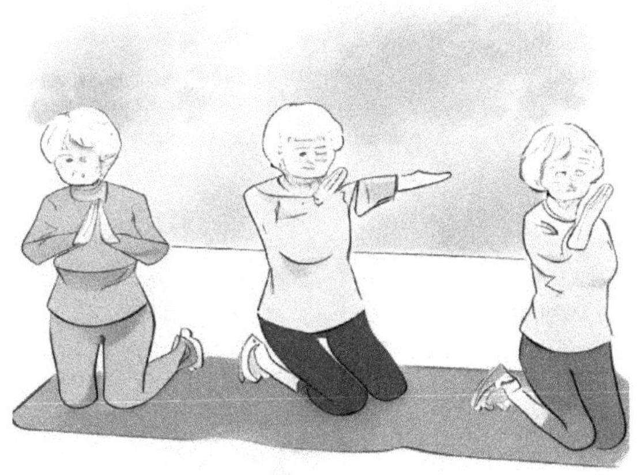

Motivational Exercise Quote

Every step you take today is an investment in your tomorrows.

Stay active, stay young at heart.

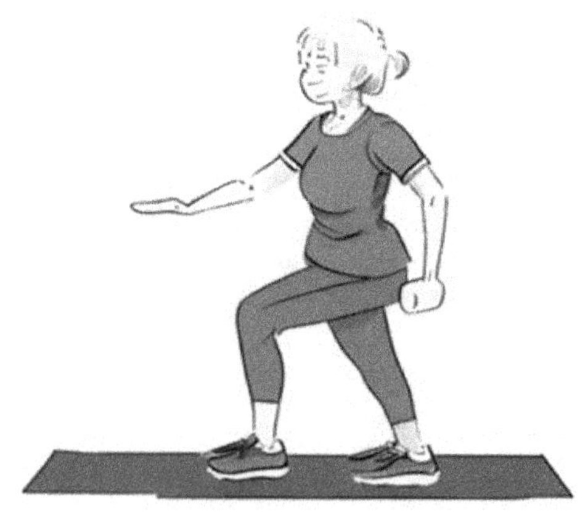

CHAPTER 3

TYPES OF CORE EXERCISES FOR SENIORS EXPLAINED IN DETAILS

I. Core Exercise while seated

Seated core exercises are exercises that focus on strengthening the core muscles while sitting. These exercises target the abdominal muscles, obliques, lower back, and hip flexors.

Core muscles are responsible for stabilizing the torso and spine, and are essential for performing everyday activities like sitting, standing, and lifting.

Seated core exercises can be used to improve posture, reduce back pain, and prevent injury.

Common seated core exercises include:

-Seated Abdominal Crunches: Sit up straight on the floor with your knees bent and feet flat on the ground.

Lean back a little and put your hands behind your head. Engage your core muscles and lift your shoulders off the floor. Hold this position for a few seconds before slowly lowering your shoulders back down.

-Seated Oblique Twists: With your knees bent and your feet flat on the floor, sit up straight. Lean back a little and put your hands behind your head.

Engage your obliques and twist your torso to the left, bringing your right shoulder across your body towards your left knee.

Hold this posture for some seconds before resuming your original position gradually. Repeat on the other side.

-Seated Leg Raises: Sit up straight on the floor with your knees bent and feet flat on the ground. Lean back a little and put your hands behind your head. Engage your core muscles and lift your legs straight off the ground until they are parallel to the floor. Before dropping your legs back down gradually, hold this posture for a couple of seconds.

-Seated Knee Tucks: Sit up straight on the floor with your knees bent and feet flat on the ground. Lean back a bit and put both hands behind your head.

Engage your core muscles and bring your knees up towards your chest. Maintain this posture for a short while before resuming your original position gently.

Seated core exercises can be used to improve core strength and stability, and are an effective way to work the core without having to stand up. They can be performed at home, in the office, or even on the go.

II. Mat Core Exercise

Mat Core exercises are exercises that focus on strengthening the core muscles. These muscles include the abdominals, obliques, and lower back muscles.

Mat core exercises typically involve using body weight and gravity to target the core muscles.

The most common mat core exercises include:

Planks, crunches, bridges, and leg lifts.

Planks are a fantastic workout for the core muscles.

They involve holding a plank position for a certain amount of time while keeping the body in a straight line.

To do a plank, start on the ground on all fours, then move into a push-up position with your arms straight and your feet together. Keep your body in a straight line and hold the position for as long as you can.

Crunches are another exercise that target the core muscles. To begin a crunch, lie on your back on the floor with your knees bent and your feet flat.

Put your hands behind your head and then curl your body up towards your knees, engaging your core muscles throughout the movement.

Bridges are a great way to work the core muscles. To do a bridge, start by lying on your back on the floor with your feet flat and your knees bent.

Lift your hips off the ground and press your feet into the ground to lift your body up. Hold the position for a few seconds, then bring your body back down.

Leg lifts are another exercise that target the core muscles. To do a leg lift, start by lying on your back on the floor with your legs straight up towards the ceiling.

Lift one leg up towards the ceiling and hold for a few seconds, then lower it back down. Repeat with the other leg.

Mat core exercises are an effective way to strengthen the core muscles. They may be done anywhere and don't need any special equipment.

These exercises can be done on their own or added to other exercises to make them more challenging.

Doing mat core exercises regularly will help to improve overall core strength and stability.

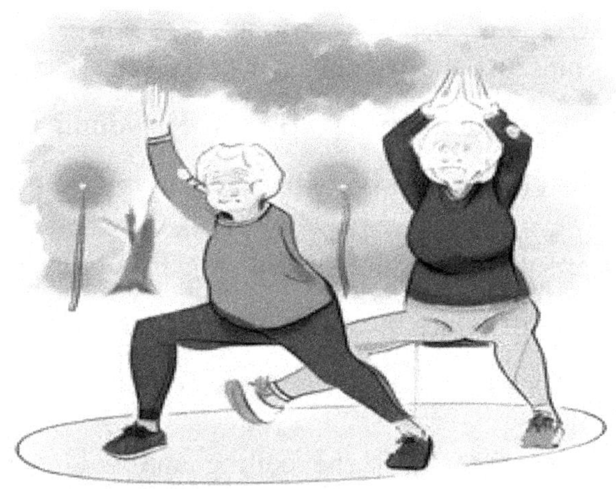

III. Walking Core Exercise

Walking core exercise is a type of exercise that focuses on strengthening the core muscles of the body, which include the abdominal muscles, the back muscles, and the hips.

The core muscles are important for maintaining balance and posture, as well as providing stability for other movements.

The goal of walking core exercises is to improve core strength, stability, and range of motion. Steps on how to engage in a walking exercise.

To do a walking core exercise, start by:

Keeping your feet shoulder-width apart while standing upright.

Engage your core muscles by contracting your abdominal muscles and drawing your belly button in towards your spine.

Keep your back straight and chest lifted. Begin walking forward, taking small steps while keeping your core engaged throughout the movement.

Make sure that your feet stay flat on the ground and don't lift your heels off the ground. Make sure to keep your core engaged and contract your abdominal muscles as you walk.

You can make this exercise more challenging by adding movement as you walk. For example, you can add arm movements such as swinging your arms side to side, or you can add side-to-side steps.

You can also increase the speed at which you walk. Additionally, you can add weight such as a medicine ball to make the exercise more challenging.

Walking core exercises can be done anywhere and are a great way to strengthen your core muscles and improve your overall balance and posture.

These exercises can be done as part of a larger workout routine or as a stand-alone exercise.

Make sure to always keep your core engaged and your back straight and chest lifted.

Start with small steps and increase the difficulty as you become more comfortable with the exercise.

IV. Standing Core Exercise

Standing core exercise is a form of exercise that focuses on strengthening the core muscles, which are the muscles located in the abdominal region and the lower back.

This type of exercise is typically performed while standing and is great for improving posture, balance, and stability.

The core muscles are important in stabilizing the spine and trunk, and they can help to reduce the risk of back pain.

Standing core exercises can help to strengthen the core muscles, which can then improve posture and balance.

How to perform a standing core exercise

1. To begin, place your feet slightly wider than hip width apart. Maintain a tiny bend in your knees and a straight back.

   Next, contract your abdominal muscles and slowly lift your arms up to the sides and out in front of your body.

   Hold this position for a few seconds, then slowly lower your arms back to your sides. This exercise should be done 8 to 10 times.

2. Another standing core exercise is the standing crunch. Start by standing with your feet hip-width apart, then slowly bend your knees and contract your abdominal muscles. Lean forward slightly and raise your arms up to shoulder height. Hold this position for a few seconds, then slowly raise your arms back up to shoulder height. Repeat this exercise 8 to 10 times.

3. Finally, the standing side plank is a great exercise for targeting the core muscles.

To perform this exercise, start by standing with your feet slightly wider than hip-width apart.

Your knees should be slightly bent while you tighten your abs.

Raise your arms up to the sides and out in front of your body. Slowly lean to one side and reach one arm up to the ceiling.

After a little period of holding this position, progressively return to your starting position. 8 to 10 times on both sides, repeat this exercise.

Standing core exercises can help to improve posture, balance, and stability.

They can also help to strengthen the core muscles, which can then reduce the risk of back pain.

A doctor should be consulted before commencing any new workout program.

Motivational Exercise Quote

Don't let age dictate your
limitations;

Let your passion for a healthier
life lead the way.

CHAPTER 4

VITAL CORE EXERCISES ROUTINE YOU SHOULD NEVER NEGLECT

Are you a senior over 60 looking for a vital core exercise routine that you should never neglect? Look no further. These core exercises routine are specifically designed to help seniors maintain their core strength, stability, and balance.

This vital routine will help you to improve your posture, reduce the risk of falls, and even improve your overall mobility.

The Core exercise routine you should never neglect include:

1. **Pain and Aches routine**

Pain and Aches Routine As we age, our bodies start to ache and cause us pain. This pain can be caused by a variety of different things, such as an injury, arthritis, or just plain old age.

Regardless of the cause, pain and aches can make it difficult to stay active and enjoy life. Fortunately, there are exercises that can help alleviate the pain and aches that come with age.

The pain and ache routine are specifically designed to reduce pain and discomfort associated with aging.

The routine consists of a number of exercises that target the core muscles, as well as other muscles in the body. By strengthening the core muscles and other muscles in the body, the routine helps to reduce pain and aches.

The routine begins with a warm-up, which helps to get the blood flowing and the muscles ready for the workout.

During the warm-up, some of the exercises that are included are stretching, walking, jogging, and using an elliptical machine. After the warm-up, the routine moves into the core exercises.

The core exercises that are included in the routine focus on strengthening the core muscles.

This includes exercises such as planks, squats, and lunges. These exercises help to strengthen the core and reduce pain and aches.

After the core exercises are completed, the routine moves into the stretching exercises. These exercises help to improve flexibility and reduce pain and aches.

Some of the stretching exercises that are included in the routine are hamstring stretches, quadriceps stretches, and calf stretches.

Finally, the routine ends with some relaxation exercises. These exercises help to reduce tension and stress, which can lead to increased pain and aches.

Some of the relaxation exercises that are included in the routine are deep breathing, progressive muscle relaxation, and visualization. The pain and aches routine is an excellent routine for seniors over 60.

It helps to reduce pain and aches, while also strengthening the core muscles and improving flexibility.

By doing this routine on a regular basis, seniors can enjoy a more active and pain-free lifestyle.

2.   Active well-being routine

Active living routines are an important part of staying healthy, especially as we age. Engaging in a regular routine of physical activity helps to maintain muscle strength, balance, and coordination, all of which are essential for maintaining our independence and quality of life.

For those over the age of 60, there are certain activities that should be included in an active living routine. These activities can range from low impact exercises like walking or swimming to more strenuous activities like strength training.

All of these activities should be tailored to each individual's fitness level and health goals. A good active living routine includes aerobic exercise.

This type of exercise strengthens the heart, lungs, and circulatory system and helps to burn calories and reduce body fat.

Aerobic exercises can include walking, jogging, swimming, cycling, and using an elliptical machine. To get the most out of aerobic exercise, it is important to maintain an intensity level that is challenging but not too strenuous.

Strength training is another important component of an active living routine. Strength training helps to build and maintain muscle mass, which is essential for maintaining an independent lifestyle.

Strength training exercises can include using weights, resistance bands, body weight exercises, and Pilates. It is important to focus on all major muscle groups, including the chest, back, shoulders, arms, legs, and core.

Stretching and flexibility exercises are also important for an active living routine. Stretching helps to improve range of motion and reduce the risk of injury.

Flexibility exercises can include yoga and tai chi. Balance exercises are also essential for an active living routine. Balance exercises help to improve coordination and reduce the risk of falls. Balance exercises can include standing on one foot, walking heel to toe, and marching in place.

Finally, it is important to include activities that are enjoyable and motivating. These can include dancing, gardening, playing sports, and even playing with grandchildren.

Anything that incorporates movement and gets the heart rate up is beneficial to an active living routine. An active living routine is essential for seniors to maintain independence and quality of life.

By incorporating a mixture of different activities into their routine, seniors can stay active and healthy well into their golden years.

3.   Within the house routine

The importance of core exercises for seniors over 60 cannot be understated. A strong core helps improve balance, posture, and overall agility. It can help reduce the risk of falls, improve digestion, and reduce the risk of back pain.

A strong core also helps with activities of daily living, such as getting in and out of bed, getting dressed, and even walking.

So, for those who are unable to make it to the gym, or if you simply prefer to exercise at home, there are plenty of core exercises you can do right in your own living room.

Here is a comprehensive list of exercises that can be easily implemented into a routine that you can do while you are at home.

One of the most basic core exercises to start with at home is **the plank**.

This exercise works your entire core, as well as your arms and legs. To do a plank, begin by laying on your stomach with your feet and hands flat on the ground.

Make sure your body is in a straight line from your head to your feet. You should hold this position for about 30-60 seconds.

The bridge exercise is another great core exercise to do at home.

To do this, begin by lying on your back with your knees bent and feet flat on the ground. Lift your hips off the ground and squeeze your glutes.

Try to keep your body in a straight line from your shoulders to your knees. You should hold this position for about 30-60 seconds.

Side planks are another great way to work your core at home.

To do this, begin by lying on your left side with your legs out straight and your forearm on the ground. Lift your hips off the ground and squeeze your glutes. Try to keep your body in a straight line from your head to your feet.

You should hold this position for about 30-60 seconds before switching to the other side.

Another great core exercise that you can do at home is the **mountain climber**.

To do this, begin in a plank position. Then, alternate bringing your knees up towards your chest while keeping your core tight. You should do this for about 30-60 seconds.

Finally, you can also do some core exercises while **sitting in a chair.**

To do this, begin by sitting up straight in the chair. Put your hands behind your head and pull your elbows back.

Then, tighten your core muscles and slowly lift your feet off the ground. Hold this position for about 30-60 seconds.

These are just a few of the core exercises you can do at home to help improve your balance and strengthen your core.

Remember to always consult your doctor before beginning any new exercise routine. With some dedication and consistency, you can strengthen your core and improve your overall health and vitality.

The Most Reliable Way to be Consistent with The Routine

The most reliable way to be consistent with your core exercises routine is by taking the necessary steps to make sure that you stick to your routine.

Consistency is key when it comes to core exercises; if you don't stick to your routine, then you won't get the results you want.

Here are some tips to help you stay consistent with your core exercises.

1. Set realistic goals – When creating your core exercise routine, make sure you set realistic goals for yourself. If you set goals that are too ambitious, you may become discouraged and give up. Choose a routine that you feel comfortable doing and that will help you progress.

2. Track your progress – Whether you choose to record your progress on paper or in an app, tracking your progress is a great way to stay motivated and stay on course. You can use this data to make sure you are meeting or exceeding your goals and make changes to your routine if needed.

3. Schedule it in – Scheduling your core exercises helps to ensure that you will find the time to do them. Try to set aside a specific time each day or week to do your core exercises. This will help to ensure that you never skip a session.

4. Make it enjoyable – Finding ways to make your core exercises enjoyable can help to keep you motivated.

Whether it's listening to your favorite music while you do them or having a friend join you, having something to look forward to will help you stay consistent with your routine.

5. Reward yourself – Rewarding yourself for sticking to your core exercises routine is a great way to stay on track. Create rewards for yourself that are meaningful and something to look forward to.

This could be anything from buying yourself something new, taking a day off from exercising, or treating yourself to a massage.

By following these tips, you can ensure that you stay consistent with your core exercises routine.

Setting realistic goals, tracking your progress, scheduling it in, finding ways to make it enjoyable, and rewarding yourself are all great ways to stay motivated and on track.

Consistency is key when it comes to hitting your fitness goals, so make sure you take the necessary steps to stay consistent with your core exercises.

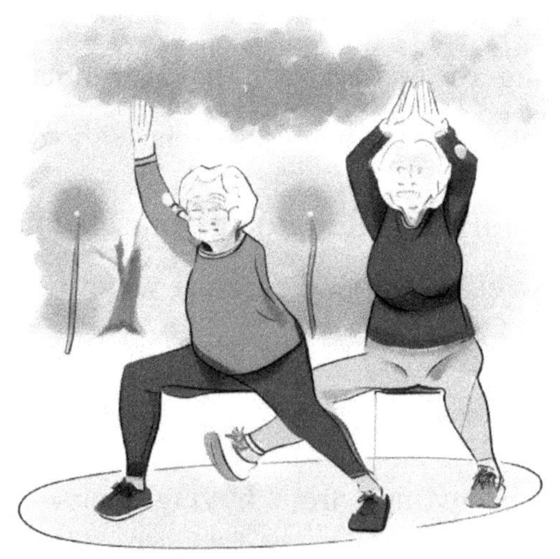

CHAPTER 5

INTERESTING CORE EXERCISES WITH YOUR PARTNER

Seniors can engage in interesting core exercises as partners to help improve their overall strength, balance, and flexibility. Partner core exercises are also a great way for seniors to socialize and have fun while exercising.

One interesting partner core exercise for seniors is the **medicine ball pass**. To do this exercise, one senior stands at a distance from their partner, holding a medicine ball. The partner standing at the distance then passes the medicine ball to the senior standing next to them.

The receiving senior then passes the medicine ball back, making sure to use good form and control their movements. This exercise works the core muscles and strengthens the arms and legs.

Another fun partner core exercise for seniors is the **plank-off**. To do this exercise, both seniors lay on their stomachs, facing each other, and place their elbows and toes on the ground.

They then lift their upper bodies off the ground, supporting their weight on their elbows and toes. The seniors then hold the plank position for as long as they can, making sure to engage their core muscles.

The partner who holds the plank for the longest amount of time wins the plank-off. Seniors can also do partner core exercises such as the wheelbarrow and the partner crunch.

For the **wheelbarrow**, one senior stand upright while the other partner holds onto their ankles and walks on their hands in front of them. The partner walking on their hands then lifts the other senior's legs up, engaging the core muscles of both seniors.

For the **partner crunch**, both seniors lie on their backs, facing each other and place their feet on the ground.

They then lift their upper bodies off the ground and touch each other's hands, crunching their abdominal muscles.

Partner core exercises are a great way for seniors to stay fit and active. Not only do they improve strength, balance, and flexibility, but they are also a great way for seniors to socialize and have fun.

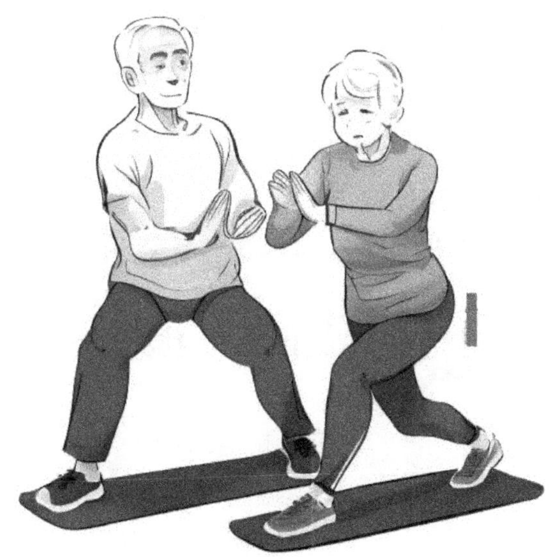

Motivational Exercise Quote

Your body is your most valuable asset

It appreciates regular deposits of movement.

Keep it active, and it will reward you with vitality.

CHAPTER 6

UNIQUE CORE EXERCISES WEEKLY SCHEDULE

WEEK 1

Monday: Core exercise 1

–**Seated twists:** Sit on a chair with your feet flat on the floor. Place your hands behind your head and twist your torso to the left and then to the right for 30 seconds each side.

Tuesday: Core exercise 2

–**Standing trunk rotations:** Stand with your feet shoulder-width apart and your arms outstretched in front of you. Rotate your torso to the left and then to the right for 30 seconds each side.

Wednesday: Core exercise 3

–Modified Push-ups: Place your hands and feet on a wall and slowly lower your body down the wall, keeping your core tight. Hold the position for 5 seconds before returning to the starting position. Repeat 10 times.

Thursday: Core exercise 4

–Plank: Lie face down and prop yourself up on your forearms. Keep your core tight, hold for 10 seconds, and then lower yourself down. Repeat 10 times.

Friday: Core exercise 5

–Leg lifts: Lie on your back with your legs in the air, and then slowly lower them down. Hold the position for 5 seconds before returning to the starting position. Repeat 10 times.

Saturday: Core exercise 6

–Bird dogs: Get on all fours. Lift your right arm and left leg at the same time and hold the position for 5 seconds. Then switch sides and repeat 10 times.

WEEK 2

Monday: Core exercise 7

–Superman: Lie on your stomach and raise your arms and legs off the ground. Hold for 5 seconds and then lower your arms and legs. Repeat 10 times.

Tuesday: Core exercise 8

–Side plank: Lie on your side and prop yourself up on your forearm. Keep your core tight, hold for 10 seconds, and then lower yourself down. Repeat 10 times.

Wednesday: Core exercise 9

–Reverse crunches: Lie on your back with your legs in the air, and then slowly crunch your legs up towards your chest. Hold the position for 5 seconds before returning to the starting position. Repeat 10 times.

Thursday: Core exercise 10

–Mountain climbers: Get on all fours and alternate bringing your knees to your chest for 30 seconds.

Friday: Core exercise 11

–Glute bridges: Lie on your back with your knees bent and feet flat on the floor. Raise your hips off the ground and hold for 5 seconds before returning to the starting position. Repeat 10 times.

Saturday: Core exercise 12

–Plank jacks: Get into a plank position and jump your legs out and in while keeping your core tight. Repeat 30 times.

WEEK 3

Monday: Core exercise 13

–Seated rows: Sit on a chair with your feet flat on the floor and a towel under your feet. Pull the towel with your arms and hold for 5 seconds before returning to the starting position. Repeat 10 times.

Tuesday: Core exercise 14

–Bicycle crunches: Lie on your back with your hands behind your head and your legs in the air. Simulate a bicycle ride by alternating twisting your torso and legs. Repeat 30 times.

Wednesday: Core exercise 15

–Leg raises: Lie on your back with your legs in the air and then slowly raise your legs up and down. Hold the position for 5 seconds before returning to the starting position. Repeat 10 times.

Thursday: Core exercise 16

–Squats: Stand with your feet shoulder-width apart and slowly lower your body down until your thighs are parallel to the floor. Hold the position for 5 seconds before returning to the starting position. Repeat 10 times.

Friday: Core exercise 17

–   Plank walk: Get into a plank position and walk your hands and feet out to the sides and then back to the starting position. Repeat 10 times.

Saturday: Core exercise 18

–Toe taps: Lie on your back and raise your legs off the ground. Slowly tap your toes to the ground and then lift them back up. Repeat 30 times.

WEEK 4

Monday: Core exercise 19

–Plank hold: Get into a plank position and hold for 10 seconds. Repeat 10 times.

Tuesday: Core exercise 20

–Reverse plank: Sit on the ground with your feet flat on the floor and your palms on the ground behind you. Raise your hips off the ground and hold for 5 seconds before returning to the starting position. Repeat 10 times.

Wednesday: Core exercise 21

–Seated twists: Sit on a chair with your feet flat on the floor. Place your hands behind your head and twist your torso to the left and then to the right for 30 seconds each side.

Thursday: Core exercise 22

–Standing trunk rotations: Stand with your feet shoulder-width apart and your arms outstretched in front of you. Rotate your torso to the left and then to the right for 30 seconds each side.

Friday: Core exercise 23

–Bird dogs: Get on all fours. Lift your right arm and left leg at the same time and hold the position for 5 seconds. Then switch sides and repeat 10 times.

Saturday: Core exercise 24

–Abdominal crunches: Lie on your back with your knees bent and feet flat on the floor. Place your hands behind your head and slowly crunch your upper body up towards your knees. Hold the position for 5 seconds before returning to the starting position. Repeat 10 times.

There is a core exercise planner just before the concluding part of this book, where you can record your fitness progress.

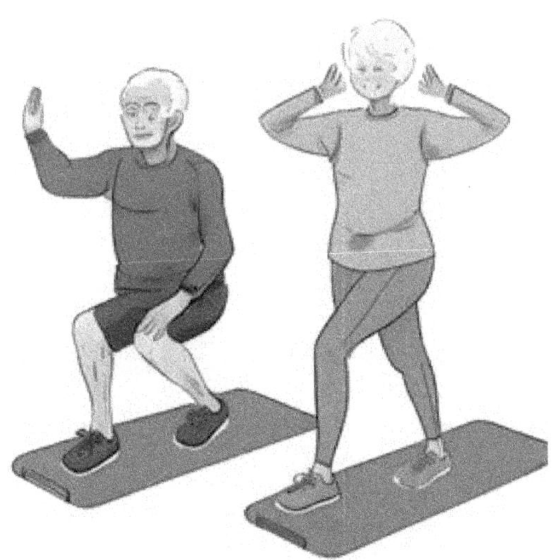

Motivational Exercise Quote

Exercise isn't about being the best;

It's about being better than you

were yesterday.

Embrace progress, not perfection

CHAPTER 7

THE MOST IMPORTANT STRETCHING AND MOBILITY EXERCISES FOR SENIORS

Stretching and mobility exercises are an important part of staying healthy and fit, especially for seniors over 60.

Not only can they help maintain muscle strength and flexibility, but they can also reduce the risk of injury, improve balance, and reduce joint pain. Additionally, these exercises can help increase independence and make day-to-day activities easier to manage.

In this chapter, we will discuss the importance of stretching and mobility exercises, tips for getting started, and some specific stretches and mobility exercises seniors can do to stay active and healthy.

The Benefits of Stretching and Mobility Exercises

Stretching and mobility exercises provide many benefits for seniors over 60. By increasing flexibility and range of motion, seniors can perform everyday activities more easily and with less risk of injury.

Additionally, regular stretching can improve posture, reduce joint pain, reduce the risk of falls, and improve balance.

Finally, these exercises can help reduce muscle tension and stiffness, which can lead to improved sleep and an overall sense of relaxation.

Tips for Getting Started

When starting a stretching and mobility program, it is important to start slowly and to work up to more challenging exercises over time.

Make sure to check with your doctor before starting any exercise program.

It is also important to warm up before doing any stretching or mobility exercises. This can help increase blood flow to the muscles and reduce the risk of injury.

When stretching, it is important to focus on breathing deeply and to hold each stretch for 15-30 seconds.

Finally, it is important to listen to your body and stop if you feel any pain. Specific Stretches and Mobility Exercises.

The following stretches and mobility exercises can help seniors over 60 stay active and healthy:

1. Neck Rotations: Slowly rotate your neck in a circular motion in both clockwise and counter-clockwise directions.

2. Shoulder Rolls: Roll your shoulders forward and backward in a circular motion.

3. Arm Circles: Lift both arms out to the side and make small circles in both directions.

4. Lower Back Stretch: Sit on the floor with your legs straight out in front of you. Bend your right knee and place your right foot on the floor, then reach your left arm over your right leg. Hold for 15-30 seconds and switch sides.

5. Calf Raises: Stand with your feet shoulder-width apart and slowly raise up onto your toes. Hold for a few seconds before slowly lowering your heels back to the floor.

6. Hamstring Stretch: Lie on your back and bring your right knee up to your chest. Use your hands to grab your right shin and gently pull your leg closer to your chest.

Hold for 15-30 seconds and switch sides.

Stretching and mobility exercises can help seniors over 60 stay active and healthy. Not only can they increase flexibility and range of motion, but they can also reduce the risk of injury, improve balance, and reduce joint pain.

Make sure to check with your doctor before starting any exercise program, and be sure to warm up before doing any exercises.

Finally, focus on breathing deeply and listening to your body while performing any stretches or mobility exercises.

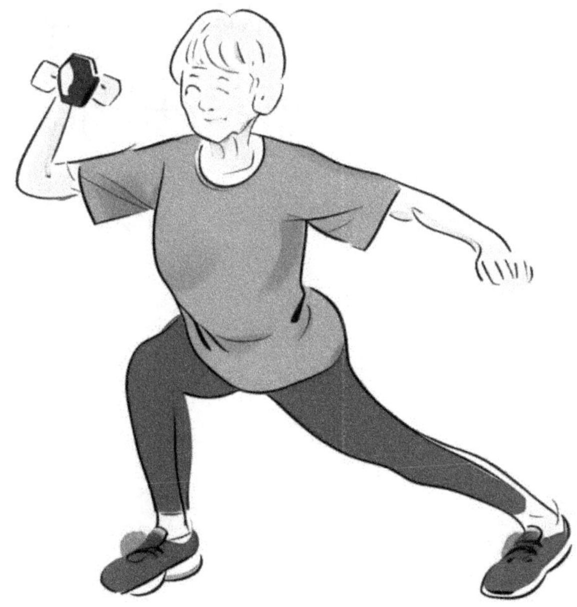

Motivational Exercise Quote

The journey of a thousand miles begins with a single step.

Start small, but start today, and watch your strength grow.

CHAPTER 8

PERTINENT SAFETY CONSIDERATIONS FOR CORE EXERCISES YOU MUST FOLLOW

Safety is a top priority when it comes to engaging in physical activity, and core exercises are no exception.

Core exercises are important for strengthening the muscles of the abdomen, obliques, and lower back, and they can provide a great benefit to overall fitness and health.

However, it is important to consider the safety considerations associated with core exercises before engaging in them.

First and foremost, it is important to ensure that you are using proper form when performing core exercises. Failure to do so can lead to injury, particularly in the lower back.

When performing any core exercise, make sure you are aware of your posture, and keep your spine in a straight line. Additionally, be sure to keep your abdominal muscles engaged throughout the exercise to ensure proper core stability.

Second, it is important to select the appropriate level of intensity for your core exercises.

If you are new to exercise, it is best to start out with lighter exercises and gradually increase the intensity as you become more comfortable with the movements. Additionally, it is important to warm up your core muscles with stretching and dynamic exercises before engaging in any core exercises.

Lastly, it is important to listen to your body when engaging in core exercises.

If you experience any pain or discomfort, stop the exercise and consult with a medical professional before continuing. Additionally, be aware of your hydration and nutrition levels before engaging in core exercises, as these can have an impact on your performance and safety.

Safety should always be a top priority when engaging in core exercises. It is important to ensure proper form, select the appropriate level of intensity, and listen to your body to reduce the risk of injury.

Following these guidelines can help ensure that your core exercises are safe and effective.

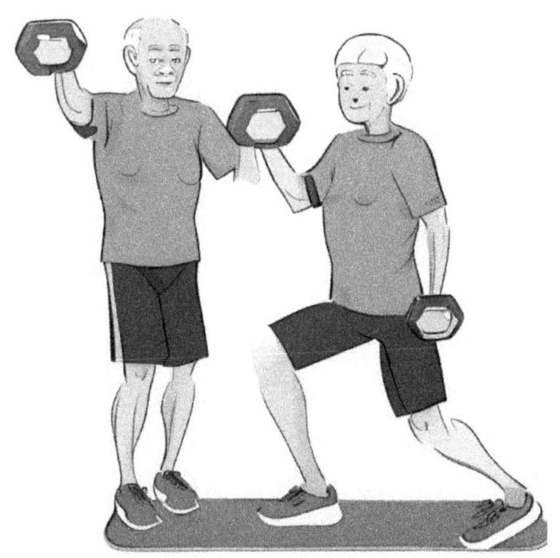

Motivational Exercise Quote

The best project you'll ever work on
is you.

Stay committed, stay active, and
create the masterpiece of your own
longevity.

CORE EXERCISE PLANNER

Core Exercise Planner

Date   Month   Year

Day	Exercise	Goal
Monday		
Tuesday		
Wednesday		
Thursday		
Friday		
Saturday		

Motivation	Notes

Core Exercise Planner

Date   Month   Year

Day	Exercise	Goal
Monday		
Tuesday		
Wednesday		
Thursday		
Friday		
Saturday		

Motivation	Notes

Core Exercise Planner

Date   Month   Year

Day	Exercise	Goal
Monday		
Tuesday		
Wednesday		
Thursday		
Friday		
Saturday		

Motivation	Notes

Core Exercise Planner

Date   Month   Year

Day	Exercise	Goal
Monday		
Tuesday		
Wednesday		
Thursday		
Friday		
Saturday		

Motivation	Notes

Core Exercise Planner

Date   Month   Year

Day	Exercise	Goal
Monday		
Tuesday		
Wednesday		
Thursday		
Friday		
Saturday		

Motivation	Notes

Core Exercise Planner

Date   Month   Year

Day	Exercise	Goal
Monday		
Tuesday		
Wednesday		
Thursday		
Friday		
Saturday		

Motivation	Notes

Core Exercise Planner

Date   Month   Year

Day	Exercise	Goal
Monday		
Tuesday		
Wednesday		
Thursday		
Friday		
Saturday		

Motivation	Notes

Core Exercise Planner

Date ________ Month ________ Year ________

Day	Exercise	Goal
Monday		
Tuesday		
Wednesday		
Thursday		
Friday		
Saturday		

Motivation	Notes

CONCLUSION

"Core exercises for seniors over 60" is an invaluable resource for anyone looking to stay healthy and active.

Staying physically fit is essential for health and quality of life, especially as we age.

Core exercises are an excellent way to remain physically fit, as they target the muscles that are essential for maintaining balance, stability, and strength.

Through this book, seniors can learn the proper techniques for performing core exercises, find exercises that are tailored to their specific needs, and discover ways to make the exercises fun and engaging.

By implementing these exercises into their daily lives, seniors can stay healthy and active, while also improving their overall quality of life.

Aging is inevitable, but embracing a vibrant life is a choice.

Let each exercise be a celebration of your strength and resilience.

LETTER TO THE READER

Dear Reader,

I am glad that you have opted to delve into the realm of health and fitness with ***"Core Exercises for Seniors Over 60".***

As a Fitness expert, I put in a lot of effort to make a book that gives you not only the exercises to advance your health, but also the wisdom to make judicious fitness decisions.

If you have any queries or comments concerning this book, please don't be hesitant to get in touch with me at **doctorbrendagrimm@gmail.com**

I'm always delighted to connect with readers and give assistance on their fitness voyage.

Sincerely,

Brenda Grimm

www.ingramcontent.com/pod-product-compliance
Lightning Source LLC
Chambersburg PA
CBHW070817280726
48660CB00016B/2057